101

ESSENTIAL TIPS

Yoga

101

ESSENTIAL TIPS

Yoga

Produced for DK by
Sands Publishing Solutions
4 Jenner Way, Eccles, Aylesford, Kent ME20 7SQ

Editorial Partners David & Sylvia Tombesi-Walton
Design Partner Simon Murrell

Senior Editor Chauney Dunford
Senior Art Editor Elaine Hewson
Managing Editor Penny Warren
Jacket Designer Kathryn Wilding
Senior Pre-production Producer Tony Phipps
Senior Producer Ché Creasey
Art Director Jane Bull
Publisher Mary Ling

Consultant Poggy Hatton

If you are pregnant or have an injury or other health concern,
consult a health professional before practising yoga.

First published in Great Britain in 2015 by
Dorling Kindersley Limited, 80 Strand, London WC2R 0RL

A Penguin Random House Company

4 6 8 10 9 7 5

008–274503–May/2015

A CIP catalogue record for this book is available from the British Library.

ISBN 978-0-2410-1476-9

Printed and bound in China

A WORLD OF IDEAS:
SEE ALL THERE IS TO KNOW

www.dk.com

101 ESSENTIAL TIPS

Pages 8 to 19
YOGA & YOU

1 ....What is yoga?
2 ....Beneficial exercise
3 ....Correct breathing
4 ....Complete relaxation
5 ....Balanced diet
6 ....Positive thinking
7 ....Increasing vitality
8 ....Nurturing the nervous system
9 ....Healthy eating
10 ....Avoid alcohol
11 ....Don't smoke
12 ....Care for your back
13 ....Energize your spine
14 ....Aligning your body
15 ....Balance both sides
16 ....Yoga for the young

17 ....Yoga for the pregnant
18 ....Yoga for the elderly
19 ....Yoga for stress
20 ....Yoga for relaxation
21 ....When to practise yoga
22 ....Where to practise yoga
23 ....Yoga classes
24 ....Yoga at home

Pages 20 to 29

GETTING STARTED

25	............................Know your body
26	.................Understand your limits
27	............................Consult a doctor
28	......................Essential equipment
29	................................What to wear
30	.........................Plan your sessions
31	.........................Keep a yoga diary
32	.................Monitor your progress
33	................................Simplify poses
34	Using props for standing positions
35	...........Using props for floor poses
36	....................Abdominal breathing
37	.................How to inhale & exhale
38	.....The importance of warming up
39	..................................Eye warm-up
40	..............................Neck warm-up
41	.......................Shoulder warm-up
42	............................Torso warm-up
43	................................Hip warm-up
44	...............................Knee warm-up
45	............................Ankle warm-up
46	................................Foot warm-up

Pages 30 to 43

POSES FOR STRENGTH

47	........How yoga improves strength
48	.............................Mountain Pose
49	....Plank
50	....Leg Raise
51	....................................Leg Raise 2
52	....Triangle
53	....Warrior
54	..............................Warrior Lunge
55	....................................Warrior 2
56	..............Downwards Facing Dog
57	...................Extended Side Stretch
58	.........................Half Spinal Twist
59	....Horse
60	....Cobra
61	......Purpose of the Sun Salutation
62	...............................Sun Salutation

Pages 44 to 53
POSES FOR TONE & STRETCH

63	....How yoga improves body tone
64	............Standing Forwards Bend
65	...............Legs Up the Wall Pose
66	...............................Bridge Pose
67	....Cobbler
68	.............Sitting Forwards Stretch
69	.............Extended Sitting Stretch
70	....................................Cat Pose
71	...............................Lunge Twist
72	................Seated Forwards Bend
73	Seated Forwards Bend Variation

Pages 54 to 59
POSES FOR RELAXATION

74	....How yoga promotes relaxation & harmony
75	..................................Cow Arms
76	...............................Child's Pose
77	..............Standing Arm Stretches
78	.........................Easy Floor Twist
79	..................................Chair Twist
80	.......Crossed Leg Forwards Bend

Pages 60 to 63
POSES FOR BALANCE

81	.........How yoga improves balance
82	......................................Tree Pose
83	...........................Half Lotus Tree
84	....Eagle
85	.....Half Shoulder Stand with Wall
86	...................................Cat Balance

Pages 64 to 69
THE COOL-DOWN

87	......Importance of the cool-down
88	........................Physical relaxation
89	..........................Mental relaxation
90	..................How long to relax for?
91	...............Ending your cool-down
92	..........................Cupping the eyes
93	....Importance of the Corpse Pose
94	..................................Corpse Pose
95	Corpse Pose: additional relaxation
96	..........................Using meditation
97	.....................What is meditation?
98	..........Where & when to meditate
99	.....................Meditation position
100	............................Yogic breathing
101	.............................Hand positions

Index 70

Acknowledgments 72

YOGA & YOU

1 WHAT IS YOGA?

The word "yoga" means "union". Yoga is a form of exercise based on the belief that the body and breath are intimately connected with the mind. By controlling the breath and holding the body in steady poses, or asanas, yoga creates harmony. Yoga consists of five key elements: beneficial exercise, correct breathing, complete relaxation, balanced diet, and positive thinking. The asanas help ease tension, tone internal organs, and improve flexibility.

UNLEASHING YOUR POTENTIAL
Yoga helps create a flexible body coupled with a relaxed but focused mental state, able to tap into the full depths of its potential.

DIG DEEP
To maximize the benefits of yoga practice, hold postures steady for several breaths, reaching for a deeper stretch on each.

2 BENEFICIAL EXERCISE

The aim of yoga practice is to improve suppleness and strength. Each posture is performed slowly in fluid movements. Jerky movements should be avoided, because they produce a build-up of lactic acid, which causes fatigue. It is also important to take into account your existing fitness and stamina. Yoga postures can be modified to make them safe for people of all abilities.

Focus in on steady, rhythmic breathing

Feel expansion and contraction of abdomen

3 CORRECT BREATHING

Yogic breathing techniques maximize oxygen levels in your blood. Correct breathing is achieved through proper execution of the asanas, so be aware of the position of your chest, ensuring that you are connecting to the movement of the diaphragm. Deep exhalations also force stale air from the lungs, and breath control facilitates the calming of, and greater ability to focus, the mind.

4 COMPLETE RELAXATION

It is most beneficial to begin and end each yoga session with relaxation. You should also take a little time to relax between asanas. Relaxation sequences apply pressure to those areas of the body that are tense, massaging them in a similar way to acupressure to release the tension held there.

ABSOLUTE MINIMUM
The yoga definition of true relaxation is the point at which the body consumes the minimum amount of energy required to exist.

Keep head facing forwards, with neck straight

Arms flat on the floor, palms up

Allow hips to fall open

Shoulders should be relaxed and flat

5 BALANCED DIET

The recommended yogic diet is very much in line with current ideas about healthy eating. It is a simple, wholesome vegetarian way of eating, comprised of natural foods that are easy to digest: fresh fruit and vegetables, dairy products, nuts and pulses. It is also important to eat in moderation and only when hungry, taking time to chew food properly.

EATING HEALTHILY
As much as possible, make the healthy choice, by favouring natural fresh ingredients over processed and tinned foods.

6 POSITIVE THINKING

In yoga, much importance is placed on the value of positive thinking in sustaining mental wellbeing. Through meditation and relaxation, yoga aims to clear the mind of negativity, while at the same time using positive affirmations to increase self-esteem. Some people think this is difficult to achieve, but practising yoga will eventually bring you to a state of mental harmony and serenity.

TAPPING INTO CREATIVITY
By channelling your thoughts in a positive direction, you will be better able to unlock your creative potential.

10

7 INCREASING VITALITY

Left unchecked, toxins build up in the body, leading to lethargy. Many yoga postures massage the internal organs that are involved in the elimination of waste products. This helps flush out toxins, thereby increasing vital nourishment to the organs and making your body function far more efficiently.

8 NURTURING THE NERVOUS SYSTEM

Practising yoga can help the nervous system to release blocked energy channels and activate healing. Postures that twist or bend the neck are particularly effective for putting the body into a restorative, healing mode. This state is also activated through the relaxation brought about by yogic breathing techniques.

Palms pressed together, drawing upwards

Lengthen through torso

Foot positioned as high as possible

Hold standing leg firm

Stretch up and back, with palms facing forwards

Arch back, pushing chest forwards

Inhale while stretching upwards

Keep legs straight

HEALTHY EATING

9 Consuming the right foods is an important part of bringing the mind and body into harmony. Foods that are beneficial to us are said to be Sattvic, or pure. Impure foods that can upset our physical, emotional, or intellectual balance are identified as being in the categories Tamasic (stale or rotten) and Rajasic (stimulating); foods that fall into these categories should be avoided by those following the yogic philosophy.

Clockwise from top: Sattvic, Rajasic, and Tamasic

FOODS TO EAT
Sattvic foods include the following: cereals; fresh fruit and vegetables; natural fruit juices; dairy products such as milk, cheese and butter; beans, nuts, and pulses; honey; and pure water.

FOODS TO AVOID
Tamasic foods include: meat and fish; mushrooms; and products that have been frozen, preserved, or tinned. • Rajasic items include: onions and garlic; tobacco; eggs; coffee and tea; strong spices; and chocolate.

AVOID ALCOHOL

10 Alcohol contains fermented products, introducing toxins into the body and overexciting the mind. Consequently, it is both Tamasic and Rajasic. Improve your mental clarity and physical wellbeing by avoiding alcohol.

Remove all alcohol from your diet

DON'T SMOKE

11 Tobacco is another product that is both Rajasic and Tamasic. By giving up smoking you will eliminate toxins from your body, helping you to achieve a calm mind and body.

Say no to cigarettes

CARE FOR YOUR BACK

Yoga postures flex and extend each section of the spine to help it regain its inherent flexibility. Each of the vertebrae goes through the full range of movement in all directions, although to varying degrees depending on the pose. The increased mobility of the intervertebral discs reduces injuries, since there is less strain on movement. The postures work on toning and strengthening the muscles that support the back, giving additional support to the spine.

Turn head to right

Press elbow against knee

HALF SPINAL TWIST
The benefits of this pose (see p.39) include strengthening of the back and thighs, as well as improving your posture.

Rotate head to left

Bring left thigh over right leg

Keep left foot relaxed

EASY FLOOR TWIST
This posture (see p.57) helps relieve tension in the back. The twisting motion helps in the revitalization of the abdominal organs.

Tilt head back and look up

Broaden shoulders to open chest

COBRA
The Cobra asana (see p.41) strengthens the spine, arms, and wrists, increases spinal flexibility, and helps energize the body.

Bend spine as far as is comfortable

ENERGIZE YOUR SPINE

13

Yoga asanas flex and extend different sections of the spine to varying degrees in order to develop spinal flexibility. The poses that offer the most obvious benefits for the spine include back and forwards bends and twists. Such postures help maintain and restore the spine's support network, such as the ligaments that bind vertebrae together, spinal joints, and the discs between the vertebrae, as well as the surrounding muscles.

Cervical vertebrae allow head to pivot freely

Thoracic vertebrae extend from base of neck to bottom of ribcage

Fused sacral vertebrae connect to pelvic girdle and assist walking and running

Last five vertebrae fuse to form tailbone or coccyx, which aids balance

CORRECTING CURVATURE

Yoga poses help correct any abnormal curvatures of the spine that may have developed through poor posture.

NOURISHING THE SPINAL CORD

A flexible spine nourishes the cerebrospinal fluid that surrounds the spinal cord and allows *prana*, or vital energy, to flow freely throughout the body.

ALIGNING YOUR BODY

14 The cornerstone of yoga is learning to hold your body in line. Consider the body as a single unit that is segmented into eight parts – head, trunk, arms, forearms, hands, thighs, legs, and feet – and remember that the straight line can be horizontal, vertical, or angled, depending on the particular yoga posture you are attempting.

INTERNAL MIRROR

Try to create a mind-map, or "internal mirror", of your body. Use this to realign the body by working slowly up, from the toes to the head. Make tiny adjustments until you feel grounded and centred. Become aware of your breathing pattern as you ease into correct alignment.

Raise arms straight up, palms facing inwards

Tilt head back slightly

Inhale as you lift arms

BALANCE BOTH SIDES

15 In everyday life, many activities work or emphasize one part or side of the body. However, for balance and harmony, it is important to keep all body parts equally strong. That is why in yoga the same exercises are repeated on both sides of the body.

Stretch as far as possible on one side

Stretch to the same extent on the other side

MOUNTAIN POSE

This yoga exercise (see p.30) is perfect for helping achieve spinal alignment, as well as for improving your posture.

15

16 YOGA FOR THE YOUNG

For children, yoga is a great way to develop self-awareness, self-control, and powers of concentration. If you have kids, encourage them to join you in your yoga practice. They are likely to be flexible even if they lack stamina. However, the latter will increase with regular sessions.

COPYCAT KIDS

Children have a natural curiosity and desire to mimic, so they will probably be intrigued enough by your yoga to want to join in.

17 YOGA FOR THE PREGNANT

Practising yoga during the antenatal period can be a valuable learning experience. Also, it can help ease your pregnancy, as well as the delivery. Work slowly and gently, allowing the poses to relax and strengthen the body and to help it adjust to the changes that are happening within. However, talk to your instructor about which poses should not be attempted while pregnant.

... AND BREATHE

Yogic breathing exercises – always important – come into their own during pregnancy, helping you make the most of your breath.

YOGA FOR THE ELDERLY

18 There is no age limit for yoga, in part because it is non-competitive and you work at your own pace. Done correctly, there is no risk of injury, and regular practice helps maintain good health and mobility. Additionally, yoga stimulates circulation and reduces the effects of arthritis.

Don't let advancing years deter you

YOGA FOR STRESS

19 Many yoga asanas help relieve stress by releasing tension that has built up in your body. Breathing exercises and meditation are also helpful, since they relax the body and calm the mind. Mental tranquillity can be further encouraged by avoiding stimulants.

Calm the mind with breathing and meditation

Ease tension by relaxing the body fully

YOGA FOR RELAXATION

20 Just as relaxing the body and mind helps get you ready for your yoga practice, your regular sessions make it easier for you to maintain a relaxed state in general – and easier to achieve that relaxed state when you are feeling the stresses and strains of daily life. The warm-up exercises on pp.26–29 are a great start, but see also the poses in Chapter 5, as well as the cool-down relaxation on pp.64–65.

Yoga helps you connect to yourself

21 WHEN TO PRACTISE YOGA

Because yoga ought to be practised on an empty stomach, early mornings or evenings tend to be the best times, but you need to consider what suits you best. Morning practice awakens the body and eases stiffness by lubricating the joints and energizing the muscles. Digestion is stimulated and mental alertness is increased, ready for a productive day. Conversely, evening yoga can help counter the stresses of the day, improving the quality of your sleep. Whichever you choose, setting aside a regular time is good for establishing a routine.

22 WHERE TO PRACTISE YOGA

You don't need a special room or fancy equipment for yoga, but there are some things to consider when choosing a practice place. Ideally, opt for a private area away from distractions. If that area is spacious, even better, since this can have a positive effect on the mind and, therefore, help you relax. Try to personalize the space, too, since this can also calm the mind.

LIGHT AND AIRY
Ideally your space ought to be lit by natural light and have some form of ventilation. The floor should be level, firm, and non-slip.

OPEN-AIR YOGA
If you are lucky enough to be near a quiet, flat open space, take advantage of it. Lay down your mat, and greet the day with open-air yoga.

23 YOGA CLASSES

Regardless of how small or large your class, it is always best to have your yoga practice supervised by a qualified teacher at least until you are confident. This is the only way to learn how to ease your body correctly into and out of the asanas, as well as how to breathe correctly when holding a pose. Your teacher will also make sure you do not strain your limbs.

EXPERT HELP
Get your yoga practice off to the best possible start by taking classes. They will also help you improve your technique and build your confidence.

24 YOGA AT HOME

Yoga's portability means that, once you have some experience, you will be able to practise the postures in the comfort of your own home. Indeed, your teacher may even suggest you work at home with some of the simpler asanas or with the relaxation techniques.

MINIMAL REQUIREMENTS
With just yourself and a mat (or a comfortable floor), it is perfectly possible to practise yoga at home.

GETTING STARTED

25 KNOW YOUR BODY

Before you undertake any yoga practice, first take the time to understand your body, bearing in mind any factors that might affect its performance, such as recent surgery, pregnancy, or medical conditions.

CHECK FOR TENSION
While in an asana, check for any tension, and try to relax it with your breathing.

26 UNDERSTAND YOUR LIMITS

It is important to know what your body's limits are and not to force yourself beyond them. There is no rush; yoga is completely non-competitive. Continue your regular yoga sessions and you will find your body becomes more flexible with time.

27 CONSULT A DOCTOR

Regardless of age, yoga is perfectly appropriate for everyone. Nevertheless, as with any physical exercise, if you have any medical concerns or conditions, it is a good idea to check with your doctor before beginning a course.

Experienced yoga practitioners can execute incredible feats of contortion

Your doctor may check your blood pressure

ESSENTIAL EQUIPMENT

28 Yoga equipment will keep you safer and more comfortable while you practise. Some pieces, such as blocks and straps, can also be used to help you achieve poses that would otherwise be beyond your capabilities, as you continue to work on expanding your level of flexibility. Props and supports can also extend the time you can hold a pose with proper body alignment.

YOGA KIT CHECKLIST
The equipment you are most likely to need or find useful in your yoga practice comprises:
• Slip-resistant mat
• Block, usually foam
• Strap or belt
• Cushion
• Towel

INEXPENSIVE PASTIME
Most yoga teachers will have equipment for use in classes, but it is all affordable enough to make it worth investing in your own.

WHAT TO WEAR

29 Whatever you wear for your yoga sessions should be comfortable and must allow complete freedom of movement. Ideally, you would practise in bare feet, but socks are fine. If practical to do so, also remove any dangling jewellery before beginning your session, since it may easily distract or annoy you.

Lightweight, loose-fitting clothes

Tight, stretch-material clothes

21

PLAN YOUR SESSIONS

30 More experienced yoga practitioners working alone may find it useful to create a plan in advance of each session, or to work out what sequence of asanas they will progress through. This will save time deciding between postures.

SAMPLE WORKOUT
1. *Mountain Pose*
2. *Triangle Pose*
3. *Warrior 2*
4. *Extended Side Stretch*
5. *Downwards Facing Dog*
6. *Warrior*
7. *Warrior Lunge*
8. *Cobra*
9. *Cat Balance*
10. *Plank*
11. *Child's Pose*
12. *Cobbler*
13. *Corpse Pose*

1   2   3   4   5

6   7   8   9

10   11   12   13

KEEP A YOGA DIARY

31 Writing in a yoga diary after each session will help you track your goals and accomplishments, as well as allowing you to identify any problem areas that need more attention. A yoga diary can also act as a means of reinforcing your practice, so you can more easily tailor it to your own needs.

SET YOUR GOALS
Although yoga is not a competitive pursuit, it can be fun and rewarding to set your own goals in a yoga diary.

MONITOR YOUR PROGRESS

32 It's important when practising any discipline to have a way of tracking progress. As well as keeping a yoga diary, a good method of self-assessment is to listen to your body. This requires practice and concentration, but once you are attuned to your body, you will be able to identify the benefits of your practice.

REFLECT FOR A MOMENT
Take time to reflect on your progress. This will help you build a firm foundation for your future yoga sessions.

SIMPLIFY POSES

33 When you first start yoga, you will almost certainly experience some stiffness and soreness in the joints. This shows you are working areas that may have been neglected. Building flexibility in these parts requires patience and commitment. If you find a specific pose hard, practise a modified version until you can progress.

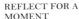

Use props such as walls and blankets to modify difficult poses

USING PROPS FOR STANDING POSITIONS

Forward bends and other standing postures may be beyond your reach to perform correctly when you first attempt them. Blocks or other means of support – a chair, for example – can be used to modify the posture so that increased flexibility can be gradually attained without injuring yourself.

Using a block to support the head

Keep back straight and in line with arms

Keep feet hip-width apart

Chair should be high enough to achieve straight line from tailbone to hands

Using a chair for additional support

USING PROPS FOR FLOOR POSES

By using a strap or a belt, you can start working towards achieving a posture that would otherwise be impossible for you when you first begin to practise yoga. When lying down, cushions and blankets can help provide the comfort you need in order to relax fully.

Hold ends of strap with both hands

Using a strap

Supports can be used to reduce discomfort

Using a cushion and a folded blanket

ABDOMINAL BREATHING

36 It is important to learn how to breathe efficiently for yoga. Lying on your back, place your hands either side of your navel. Feel how the abdomen expands as you inhale and contracts as you exhale. By breathing slowly and deeply, you are able to take air into the lowest parts of your lungs, while also exercising your diaphragm.

Hands separate slightly as abdomen expands

Fingers touch as abdomen contracts

Inhalation

Exhalation

HOW TO INHALE & EXHALE

37 Inhalation can be used to lengthen and expand within an asana, while exhalation helps release deeper into the pose. Careful and progressive work within postures will allow for a full, easy-flowing breath, which is a crucial indicator of how well the asana is being executed. In this respect, the breath and asana practice must work together.

Shoulders move up slightly

Chest expands up and out

Let belly expand as diaphragm contracts

Chest moves down

As diaphragm relaxes, navel is drawn in

Inhalation

Exhalation

38 THE IMPORTANCE OF WARMING UP

Before beginning a yoga session, make sure you are fully warmed up. Carry out the exercises shown in Tips 39–46. You should also take some time to practise your breathing techniques (see Tips 36 and 37). Mastering breath control will allow you to breathe more deeply, enable you to position yourself correctly in the yoga asanas, and assist you in holding the poses.

39 EYE WARM-UP

This series of exercises is purely for the eyes, so be sure not to move the head or neck while doing them. Look up (below left). Look right (below middle left). Look up diagonally to the right (middle right). Look down (right). Repeat the sequence, this time looking to the left side and up diagonally to the left. Hold each position for a few seconds.

Looking up

Looking right

Looking up and right

Looking down

40 NECK WARM-UP

Sit upright with your back straight. Slowly tilt your head forwards, and then backwards. Then tilt your head to the right, before repeating the same to the left. Finally, rotate your head 90 degrees to the right and then again to the left side. Hold each position for a few seconds. Never move your neck beyond what is comfortable.

Tilting head forwards

Rotating head to the right

Tilting head to the right

41 SHOULDER WARM-UP

Stand upright with your fingertips on your shoulders and your elbows out to the side. Inhale, bringing your elbows in front of you so they touch. Exhale, lifting the elbows up and apart, stretching them up. Finally, lower the elbows down. Repeat ten times.

Fingertips on shoulders

Keep shoulders level

Exhale

Bring elbows together

Lift sternum and open chest

Inhale

Stretch upper arms upwards

Elevate shoulders

Exhale

Keep neck centred

Relax shoulders

Inhale

42 TORSO WARM-UP

Start by standing with your feet hip-width apart and your palms resting on your hips. Gently and rhythmically, twist your upper body side to side, rotating at the hips, waist, and spine. Perform ten twists on each side, also allowing your head and shoulders to go with the movement.

Shoulders follow rotation movement

Hands placed on hips

Twisting to the right

Shoulders swing side to side

Twist entire upper body

Twisting to the left

HIP WARM-UP

43 Start by standing with your feet hip-width apart, and put your hands on your hips. Keeping your legs straight and kneecaps pulled up, rotate the hips in a circle, ten times clockwise and ten times anti-clockwise. Make sure you engage the hips and upper body in the roll.

Tilt torso with rotation

Keep hands on hips

Hold legs as straight as possible

Keep facing forwards, not up or down

Rotate hips in a circular motion

Rotating the hips clockwise

Rotating the hips anti-clockwise

KNEE WARM-UP

44 Stand with your feet together and with your legs slightly bent at the knees. Bring your hands to rest lightly on your kneecaps, with fingers pointing downwards. Rotate your knees gently in a circular motion, ten times in each direction, keeping your feet firmly rooted to the ground.

Rotate knees

Allow ankles to move also

Fingers point downwards

Keep feet rooted

Rotating the knees clockwise

Rotating the knees anti-clockwise

ANKLE WARM-UP

45 From a standing position, lift your right leg slightly, keeping the left leg firm. Balance yourself, then gently swing the right leg, toes pointing down. Hold for a few breaths before swapping legs. Follow this by gently rotating the right foot at the ankle – first one way, then the other. Repeat with the left foot.

Point toes downwards

Support weight with spread toes

Leg swinging, with toes pointing down

"Draw" circles with big toe

Rotating the right ankle

FOOT WARM-UP

46 The feet should be stretched in both directions. First, stretch the heels a few times. Do this by lifting the right heel up as far as possible, then lowering it. Next, roll on to the front of the right toes, curling and gently pressing them under the foot. Hold for 2–3 breaths, then repeat on the left.

Toes pressed firmly

Stretching the heel

Press gently, without excessive weight

Rolling on to the toes

POSES FOR STRENGTH

HOW YOGA IMPROVES STRENGTH

All yoga asanas improve overall strength by engaging the core muscles, as well as other muscle groups depending on the pose. The muscles work to maintain balance and poise, getting stronger by moving through a range of motions while supporting the body's weight. The key to building strength over time is consistent yoga practice. Cardiovascular strength can be enhanced by regularly including the Sun Salutation (see Tip 62) in your practice, increasing both your heart rate and blood flow.

MOUNTAIN POSE

This posture is perfect for helping you to correct spinal alignment. Start with your arms by your sides, feet hip-width apart, the sides of the legs parallel, and the toes pointing forwards and pressed into the ground.

Look straight ahead

Keep torso straight

Hold stomach in

Point fingers downwards

1 Realign your body slowly, from toes to head via ankles, knees, pelvis, chest, shoulders, and neck.

Keep neck straight

Place hands in prayer pose

Pull up backs of thighs

Tighten calf muscles

2 Bring your hands in front of your chest in prayer pose. Be sure to keep your head and neck straight.

Raise arms straight up

Tilt head back slightly

Extend from spine

Keep feet grounded

3 Breathe in and stretch the arms up, palms in, and tilt the neck up slightly. Lengthen the spine.

Release tension in shoulders

Keep spine straight

Position palms on thighs

PLANK

49

The Plank pose is an all-round strengthening posture. But it is also ideal for releasing stress in the neck, as well as for lengthening the spine.

1 Sit with your legs folded under yourself and with your toes pointing away. Put your hands on your thighs, fingers pointing forwards. Straighten your neck and back, keeping your chin parallel to the floor. Allow your breath to flow in and out easily.

Pull abdomen in towards spine

Hold knees hip-width apart

Keep soles of feet upwards

Hold arms shoulder-width apart

2 Position yourself on all fours, keeping your knees hip-width apart and directly under your hips. Your arms should be parallel to your thighs, and your back flat. Pull in your abdomen.

3 As you breathe in, extend your legs, locking your knees and elbows and keeping your body straight. Grip the mat with your toes, and push your heels back. Hold for as long as you are able, then release.

Keep knees locked

Keep arms straight

Spread fingers and root down through fingertips

LEG RAISE

50

Elevating the leg provides a strong stretch to the hamstring and calf muscles. This pose develops the flexibility and strength needed for forwards-bending poses. Begin by raising each leg three times, synchronizing each movement with your breath.

Keep head centred

Breathe from abdomen

1 Lie flat on your back with your feet together and your arms on the floor at your sides, palms down. Flex your feet slightly.

Hold leg as straight as possible

2 Inhale as you raise your left leg, then exhale as you lower it. Repeat this action for the right leg. Complete five sets of raises.

On exhalation, draw navel towards spine

Keep leg straight

LEG RAISE 2

51

In this alternative version of the Leg Raise, you draw the head towards the knee to compress the abdomen. Consequently, this particular exercise strengthens the neck, abdominal, and lumbar muscles. It also helps tone the legs.

Clasp hands over knee   *Lengthen leg*

1 Lie flat on your back. As you exhale, bend your left leg, bringing the knee into your chest. Take the knee in both hands to help press your left thigh to the abdomen.

Bring forehead towards knee

2 As you inhale, lift your head towards the knee. Then exhale, slowly lowering head, arms, and leg. Repeat with the right leg. Complete the whole exercise five times.

TRIANGLE

52

This posture is excellent for building strength in the back and core. It also helps improve the flexibility of the hip joints and opens up the chest.

Stand tall

Hold thighs firm

Keep hand placed on hip

Foot turned out 90 degrees

1 Stand with feet together and hands in prayer pose, and focus on your breathing. Jump or walk your feet 1m (3ft) apart, with toes forwards and knees locked.

2 Turn your right leg out. Inhale, and raise your arms to shoulder level with your palms facing downwards, then place your left hand on your hip. As you exhale, pivot from the hip to the right. Breathe into the stretch.

3 Exhale to bring your right arm down to rest on or behind your right leg, depending on comfort, and extend your left arm straight up. Hold the pose for several breaths. Reverse the movement to release, then repeat on the left side.

Press outer edge of foot into mat

WARRIOR

53 The Warrior asana helps strengthen the mind as well as the body. Keep the lower part of the body firmly grounded while allowing the upper body the freedom to move with control and purpose.

Press palms together

Look straight at hands

Keep head centred

Rotate left leg out slightly

Tighten leg muscles

1 Start in step 1 of the Mountain Pose (see p.30). Lengthen your spine, and breathe in a gentle rhythm.

2 Exhaling, step forwards with your right foot as far as is comfortable. Put your hands on your hips, which should face forwards, and lock your knees. Angle your left foot out to about 60 degrees.

3 Inhale deeply, bending your right knee until it is above your ankle. Raise your arms straight up, palms together. Tilt your head back, and take five breaths. Exhale to release, reversing the steps. Repeat the pose with the left leg.

Pull up through abdomen

Knee should be above ankle

Keep heel in contact with mat

54 WARRIOR LUNGE

This posture really works the quadriceps, which are the muscles at the front of your thighs, as well as gently stretching your lower back.

Point toes behind you

1 Start on all fours, with your wrists under your shoulders and your knees under your hips. Draw your navel towards the spine to flatten the back.

Lean torso forwards

2 Exhaling, bring your right foot next to your right thumb. At the same time, lean forwards at a 45-degree angle, so the right side of your abdomen is next to the right thigh.

Tilt head to look up

Extend neck

Turn toes under foot

3 Raise your torso slightly by lifting your hands, keeping the fingers pressed into the mat. Lift your left knee and turn your toes under to take the weight.

Keep neck straight and long

Create hollow in lower back

Rest hands on knee

Press down through foot

4 Lift your hands onto your right knee. Look forwards and straighten your torso. Hold for five breaths. On exhalation, release and return to all fours. Repeat on the other side.

55

WARRIOR 2

This variant of the Warrior pose helps tone the abdomen, as well as strengthening the limbs and opening the chest and shoulders. Start off in step 2 of Mountain Pose (see p.30). Focus on your breathing, and centre yourself, then jump or walk your feet out so they are about 1m (3ft) apart.

Right leg faces forwards

Left leg turned out 90 degrees

1 Breathe in, and as you do so, raise your arms up, palms down, level with your shoulders. Turn your left foot until it is pointing in the same direction as your left hand. Keep the right foot facing forwards.

Ensure arms are level

Hold chin at 90 degrees

2 Rooting yourself through the feet, bend your left knee until it is directly over the ankle. Turn your head left, and look towards your left hand. Hold for five breaths and release on inhalation. Repeat on the other side.

Pull hips downwards

Keep knee in line with ankle

56 DOWNWARDS FACING DOG

This is one of the best-known of all yoga postures, and for good reason. As well as being perfect for energizing the entire body, it also helps calm the mind and gives a strong stretch in the shoulders, hamstrings, and calves. Begin on all fours with hands shoulder-width apart and knees hip-width apart.

Draw navel towards spine on exhalation

1 Move your hands slightly ahead of your shoulders, spreading your fingers so that your middle fingers are pointing forwards.

Draw back your hips
Keep your back flat
Keep arms straight

2 Turn your toes under your feet, keeping the soles vertical to the floor, and draw your hips back towards your feet.

Bring tailbone upwards
Spread toes and root down
Keep neck relaxed

3 As you exhale, lift your knees, drawing your tailbone up. Keep the knees slightly bent and your heels off the floor.

4 Straighten your arms and legs as much as you are able, and push back into your heels. Relax your neck, and breathe evenly. Every time you exhale, lengthen your spine.

Extend your back
Be aware of movement of abdomen
Keep head in line with body
Spread fingers to reduce pressure on wrists
Stretch backs of legs
Flatten feet to floor

57 EXTENDED SIDE STRETCH

Use this posture to help tone and strengthen your legs, improve lung capacity, and stimulate the organs in the abdomen.

Extend arms fully

Turn left foot in slightly

1 Stand with your feet about 1m (3ft) apart. As you inhale, raise your arms parallel to the floor, palms down. Turn your left foot in slightly and your right foot out to 90 degrees.

Turn head right to 90 degrees

Keep knee above ankle

2 Exhale, bending your right knee until it is above your right ankle. Keeping your arms parallel to the floor, stretch them out wide, locked at the elbows. Try also to bring the right thigh parallel to the floor.

Keep hips open

3 Exhale to lean your upper body forwards, with the right forearm on your thigh. Bring your left hand into the small of your back.

Arm is in line with leg

Exhale to extend further

Keep knee at 90 degrees

Root down through right foot

4 Extend your left arm up and over the back of your left ear, palm down. Stretch from the left heel up to your left fingertips. Look up at your left arm. Inhale and straighten the front leg to release. Repeat on the other side.

HALF SPINAL TWIST

58

This pose involves a lateral twist along the complete length of the spine. It helps increase your spinal flexibility and therefore benefits overall posture. It is also useful for releasing tension throughout the body. Complete the exercise on both sides.

Draw shoulders back

Concentrate on your breathing

1 Sit with your back straight and your legs extended. Keeping your arms straight, place your palms on the mat behind you, with fingers pointing away from your body. Breathe from the abdomen.

Extend arm up

Keep looking forwards

2 Bring your right foot to the mat over your left leg, next to your left calf. As you inhale, lift your left arm straight up, palm open and fingers extended.

3 Exhale, bringing the left elbow to the outside of the right knee, palm to the right. Lift upwards from the waist, then twist until you are looking over your right shoulder. Breathe slowly from the abdomen.

Turn head 90 degrees right

59

HORSE

This pose helps strengthen the core and stretch the leg muscles. It also lengthens the spine and opens the hips, making it particularly good for combating the effects of prolonged sitting.

Arms raised to 45 degrees

Keep feet about 1m (3ft) apart

1 Start with your feet about 1m (3ft) apart and turned outwards to 45 degrees. Inhale and raise the arms 45 degrees, palms forward.

Press palms together

Lift up through waist

Feet pressed into mat

2 Firm your leg muscles, and inhale slowly, sweeping the arms up until the palms are together above the head, arms fully extended.

Hold hands in prayer pose

3 Exhale as you bend your knees, being aware of your body alignment. Lower your arms, and bring your hands into the prayer pose.

Draw tailbone and pelvis down

Knees are positioned over ankles

Push down through feet

COBRA

60 This is a face-down pose that requires you to lift the upper body, curling up and back like a cobra. By holding the posture, you tone and strengthen the muscles of the back and abdomen. It also increases the flexibility of your spine and helps relieve tension.

Relax head and neck   *Push thighs into mat*

1 Lie face down, with your forehead resting on the mat and your arms by your sides, palms up. Stretch your legs, and point your toes away from your body.

Keep backs of arms flat

2 Maintain the position of your head, but bend your arms in order to bring the palms of your hands flat on the floor, on each side of your chest.

3 Take a deep breath in, and raise your head and chest, arching the spine and pressing your shoulder blades together. Hold for five to ten breaths, then return to the starting position.

Arch back

Push down through hands

PURPOSE OF THE SUN SALUTATION

61 The Sun Salutation (see overleaf) is a graceful, fluid 12-step routine that brings together several poses to loosen up body and mind in preparation for your yoga session. The positions employed are tied into your breathing pattern, helping to instil a feeling of balance and harmony. Furthermore, the order in which the postures are put together leads to a variety of beneficial spinal movements. Once you know the routine, try to complete the Sun Salutation at least six times before each yoga session.

SUN SALUTATION

Traditionally performed to greet the rising sun, this sequence of postures helps warm the muscles, flex the spine, and synchronize the breath with the movement of the body.

Keep arms apart as they rise

Align head, neck, and back

Ensure shoulders are relaxed

Bend forward from hips

Start with hands at your sides

Bend knees slightly if necessary

1 Start in step 1 of the Mountain Pose (see p.30). As you breathe out, bring your hands up into the prayer position.

2 Inhale deeply, raising the arms, palms forwards, and bend back from the waist, pushing out your hips and keeping the legs straight.

3 Exhaling, bend forwards from the hips, and place the palms beside your feet. They stay in this position for the rest of the sequence.

4 As you breathe in, stretch your left leg backwards as far as you can, and rest your left knee on the floor. Bring your shoulder blades together, and press down through your fingertips. Arch your back by tilting your face upwards.

Stretch head upwards

Extend leg back

Stretch your foot

Press toes into mat *Do not raise or drop hips* *Keep elbows straight*

5 Hold your breath as you bring your right foot back and move onto your toes so that your entire body is in a straight, inclined line.

Keep feet together *Raise hips off mat* *Keep elbows close to body*

6 Exhale, lowering your knees to the floor and your chest straight down between your hands, touching your forehead to the mat. Keep your hips raised up.

7 Inhale, lowering your hips and extending your feet backwards. Arch your spine to look upwards, pushing your chest forwards. Keep your abdomen and legs relaxed.

Tops of feet touch floor *Relax legs and abdomen* *Arch body backwards*

Lengthen tailbone away from pelvis *Keep back as straight as possible* *Lengthen through arms*

8 Exhale and turn your toes under, raising your hips to make an inverted V-shape. Push your hips back as far as possible. Keep your back straight and heels pressed down.

ENDING THE SUN SALUTATION
The last four steps of the Sun Salutation are essentially repeats of earlier poses. From step 8, move into the position in step 4 but on the other side of the body – by bringing your left leg forwards instead of back. From this lunge posture, you then work backwards through steps 3, 2, and 1, though excluding the prayer pose.

POSES FOR TONE & STRETCH

63 HOW YOGA IMPROVES BODY TONE

In yoga, muscles are worked dynamically – that is, stretched and strengthened at the same time, which is perfect for muscle tone. Regular practice will lead to greater definition as the muscles become lean and toned. When your strength and flexibility have built up, you can make your practice even more intense by holding poses for longer or by moving more swiftly between asanas. Muscle tone can also be increased through varying the choice of postures in your yoga sessions.

64 STANDING FORWARDS BEND

The chief benefit of this asana is the intense stretch that it gives you – from the middle of your back, all the way down your legs to your heels. Once you are in the final position, hold it for several breaths, lengthening the lower back and leg muscles with each.

Hold arms at your sides

Tune in to your breathing

Stand with feet hip-width apart

Keep hands shoulder-width apart

Lengthen your midriff

Lengthen backs of legs

Draw abdomen close to legs

Lengthen hamstrings

1 Stand in step 1 of Mountain Pose (see p30). Centre yourself, and focus on your breath as you root down.

2 Inhale deeply, lock your arms at the elbow and slowly sweep them up. Tilt your head to look up at your hands.

3 Exhale, bending forwards from the hips, bringing your fingertips to the floor. Lengthen the backs of the legs and place your palms next to your feet.

LEGS UP THE WALL POSE

In this posture, the upper body is supported completely by the floor, while the wall partially supports your legs, helping their upwards extension. This is an ideal asana as preparation for more advanced inverted poses.

Position shoulder against wall

Place hands on thighs

1 Sit fully upright with your left hip and shoulder pressed against the wall. Place your palms on top of your thighs.

Use hands to help stabilize yourself

2 Place your left hand against the wall, then lean back, lowering yourself down on to your right elbow, and draw up your knees.

3 Extend your legs up the wall and keep your back flat on the floor, with your hands on your stomach. Keep your legs and heels pressed against the wall, and hold the pose for several breaths.

Keep feet relaxed

Legs should be straightened and lengthened

Let abdomen rise and fall gently

Keep your head centred

66 BRIDGE POSE

This backward-bend asana promotes relaxation and can help with the reduction of stress. It stretches the spine and the thoracic and lumbar regions, but it is also a good posture to carry out when your feet are feeling tired.

Centre your head

Bend knees completely

1 Position yourself on your back, with your knees bent and your feet flat on the floor, close to your behind. Extend your arms, palms down, alongside your body.

BRIDGE VARIATIONS
If you would like more of a challenge, these variations on the Bridge work different muscle groups.

Hold thighs parallel to floor

Angle lower legs

Hamstring stretch variation
Once in the Bridge posture, take several deep breaths. Edge your feet away from you to create a 45-degree angle to the floor with your lower legs.

Keep raised leg perpendicular to floor

Extend foot, pointing toes up

Thigh parallel to floor

Leg lift variation
From the Bridge pose, raise your left leg 90 degrees to the floor and point your foot. Take five breaths, then release on exhalation. Repeat on the right.

Push hips up to arch back

Feet are hip-width apart

2 Edge the hands to the feet and hold the heels or ankles. Keep your feet firm. Inhale, pushing your hips up and arching the spine to lift the lower back clear of the floor.

Keep head centred

Use hands to support back

Keeps legs slightly apart

3 Release your feet. Keeping your upper arms planted, place your hands as high up your back as you can. Take a few deep breaths before reversing the steps to release.

COBBLER

67

This posture is good for stress relief, since it helps release tension in the hips, legs, and lower back. Additionally, it opens up the hips and improves circulation.

Centre your head

Pull back shoulders

1 Sit with your legs straight out in front of you and hands by your sides. Bend your knees and draw your feet together, positioning them sole to sole. Keep your back straight.

Allow face to relax

Bring arms to front

2 Keeping your feet pressed together, bring your hands around and take a firm hold of them. Your head should remain centred and your spine lengthened.

Rest hands on knees

Focus on your breathing

Push knees down gently

3 On an outward breath, gently extend your knees, bringing them out and down, towards the mat, letting the hips open. Continue to elongate the spine.

4 To end, slowly move the knees up towards your chest, then run your hands up from feet to knees. Rock from side to side, feeling the stretch in your hips.

47

Position foot using both hands

1 Sit with legs extended in front of you. As you inhale, bend your right leg. Take hold of the foot, and bring the heel towards you.

68 SITTING FORWARDS STRETCH

When you need to calm your mind, this is a great go-to asana. It also stretches the hamstrings and the spine, as well as massaging the abdominal organs.

Raise arms to vertical position

2 Place the sole of the right foot against the left leg. As you inhale, lift both arms straight up, with your palms forwards.

Inhale as you lift arms

Keep head aligned with back

Bring arms forwards

3 On the outward breath, bring your arms to rest on your left shin, bending from the waist. Inhale, stretching through the spine.

4 Exhale, bringing your torso towards your extended leg. Breathe in slowly as you sit back up. Repeat on the other side.

Relax your hips

Hold foot if possible

EXTENDED SITTING STRETCH

69

By extending the spine, arms, and legs all at the same time, this posture helps prepare you for other sitting stretch poses that you might include in your session.

Look straight ahead

Toes flexed towards torso

1 Sit with your legs extended in front of you, elbows locked, and palms pressed down. Breathe in deeply to lift and expand the chest.

Raise arms with palms forward initially

Fully extend legs

2 With your back upright, inhale and lift your arms. Press the palms together, interlock the fingers, and turn the palms up. Stretch up, and hold for five breaths. Release and lower.

3 Repeat step 2, this time interlocking your fingers the less natural way, so the little finger that was on top is now underneath.

Fingers are interlocked

Keep head centred

Front view

Lengthen legs by pushing heels away from you

70

CAT POSE

As well as strengthening the lower-back muscles, the Cat gives the spine and abdominal organs a gentle massage. By stretching the back, torso, and neck, it is also a good stress-relieving asana.

Keep your back straight

Relaxed neck

Thighs at 90° to floor

1 Start on all fours, with wrists under the shoulders and knees under the hips. Point the toes away from the body. Flatten your back by drawing the navel up to the spine.

Spine curves down on inhalation

Stretch neck to look forward

2 As you breathe in, gently curve the spine down by pulling the tailbone up and pushing the chest out. Raise your chin and look up.

Back is arched

Draw down crown of head

3 Exhale, lowering the tailbone and raising the abdomen, creating an upward arch in the spine. Drop your head between your arms without exerting any downward force on it.

Abdomen is raised

Stabilize yourself through palms

71 LUNGE TWIST

Practise this asana to help tone and strengthen the muscles in the upper legs. It is also a recommended posture for improving the flexibility of the spine. Come out of step 4 after a few breaths by reversing the process, then repeat on the other side.

Head is centred

Relax your shoulders

Back is naturally curved

Spread fingers to help with stability

1 Begin on your hands and knees, with your arms shoulder-width apart and your legs hip-width apart. Look down at your fingers.

2 Inhale, extending the right leg forwards, lifting up the torso and bringing the right knee directly over the ankle. Rest your hands on your right knee.

Lengthen through spine

Press top of foot into mat

3 Keeping your feet static, inhale as you lean forwards, increasing the right-knee bend. Place your hands either side of your right foot.

Arm extended with palm open

Rotate torso

Knee brought back over ankle

4 On an out breath, push the left hand into the mat, then lift your right arm up to point at the ceiling. Look at the raised hand.

LUNGE TWIST VARIATION

In this variation on (and addition to) step 4, you bring your left elbow over and across the right knee and lower the right arm to come into the prayer pose. Turn your head to look up, until your chin is over the right shoulder. On exhalation, try to open the chest and rotate the trunk.

Hands in prayer pose

Head turned 90° from centre

72 SEATED FORWARDS BEND

Although it looks like an easy posture, when it is performed correctly, the Seated Forwards Bend can work wonders on your hamstring muscles and spine.

1 Sit with your back and arms straight, palms flat on the mat and your legs stretched out in front of you. Point your feet up, and flex the toes slightly.

SIMPLIFIED FORM
People who are not flexible enough to reach their ankles can still practise this exercise. Place a strap around the balls of both feet and bring your hands as close to your feet as you are able when bending forwards with a straight back.

2 Maintaining this posture, stretch your arms up as far as possible. They should lie next to your ears. Hold the hands with open palms forwards.

Lift chest to lengthen spine

3 Again, making sure to keep your back straight, lean forwards from the waist, and reach for your ankles with straight arms. Hold for a few breaths, then release.

Keep upper back straight

Gently hold ankles

73

SEATED FORWARDS BEND VARIATION

If you want a little extra stretch in the hamstrings and lower back, try this more difficult variation on the exercise opposite. The secure grip that the hands take on the toes helps you bring your torso further over your legs.

Correct, secure hand positions

Back, neck, and head are aligned

Keep legs lengthened and flat

Lean forwards from hips

1 Sit with your legs straight out in front of you. On an out breath, bend forwards, keeping your back straight and extending your arms. Grasp your big toes with the first two fingers on each hand, as above.

Lengthen spine by lifting through chest

2 Exhaling, bend further forwards to stretch the spine. Bend your elbows so that they help you with the forwards movement. Be sure to keep your legs straight, and maintain the grip on your toes.

3 Exhale, bending further, so the elbows come to the mat and the abdomen to the thighs. With each out breath, extend more, focusing on your toes.

Extend forward with each breath out

Bring abdomen as close to thighs as possible

POSES FOR RELAXATION

74 HOW YOGA PROMOTES RELAXATION & HARMONY

The purpose of yoga is to unite all the levels of our being, bringing about harmony of mind, body, and spirit. It serves to nourish the entire body and nervous system, through improved circulation and by balancing hormones, which in turn helps promote relaxation. Breathing exercises and meditation bring about mental and spiritual calm. All these aspects work together to create relaxation and harmony within.

75 COW ARMS

This yoga pose exercises both arms simultaneously, at the same time also enhancing upper-body flexibility and awareness of your own posture.

Clasp fingers securely

Keep head centred

Rear view

Relax your shoulders

Straighten left arm fully

Breathe rhythmically

1 Kneel, sitting on your heels, with your toes pointing backwards. Look forwards and soften the muscles of the face. Relax the shoulders as you breathe.

2 Inhale, and raise your left arm up. Work the stretch along the side of your body. Bend your right elbow so that the right hand is on your lower back, palm facing out.

3 Bend your left arm, so the hand is between your shoulders. Push the right arm higher up your back, palm still out, until you can clasp the fingers of both hands together. Pull gently. Exhale to undo, and flick your fingers to release any tension. Switch sides.

Look straight ahead

Relax your shoulders

Keep knees hip-width apart

76 CHILD'S POSE

This posture offers a useful counter-stretch to backwards bends and helps normalize the circulation. The Child's Pose can be used either to prepare for, or recover from, other poses.

Feel breath at back of ribcage

Touch mat with forehead

1 Kneel, sitting on your heels, with your big toes touching. Keep your spine straight. Clasp one wrist with the other hand.

2 Exhaling deeply, slowly move your head and chest down as far as possible, bending from the hips. Continue folding forwards until your forehead rests on the mat.

3 Unclasp your hands, and allow them to rest on the floor, palms up. Focus on your breathing. Hold this position for several minutes.

Rest forehead on cushion instead of mat

An easier option

Keep shoulders relaxed

Hold clasped hands to sternum

Allow back to curve naturally

Keep feet together

77 STANDING ARM STRETCHES

This series of postures is good for those who wish to improve the harmony between their breathing and movement. It is also valuable for the stretch it gives across the shoulders and along the spine.

1 Stand with your feet together, and interlock your fingers. Place your hands on your chest, palms down. Feel the movement of your chest as you breathe.

Extend from lower back

Pull up kneecaps

Look ahead

Keep arms straight

Inhale from abdomen

2 Breathe in, stretching out your arms, with fingers interlocked but palms now facing out. Exhale to bring your arms back to your chest.

Lock elbows

Raise arms to 45°

Keep legs straight

3 Repeat the movement in step 2, but this time extending your arms up at an angle of 45 degrees. Inhale on extension, and exhale on return.

4 With the shoulders relaxed, repeat steps 1 and 2, but this time extending your arms up and lengthening your spine. Exhaling, return to the start position. Do each stretch at least five times.

EASY FLOOR TWIST

78 This exercise is ideal for relieving tension, which it does through stretching and relaxing the spine and legs. The twisting motion across the torso also helps with the detoxification of abdominal organs.

Extend arms along floor

Legs relaxed, with knees slightly apart

Allow feet to fall open

1 Lie flat on your back. Relax your shoulders, and rest your arms beside your body, palms up.

2 Bring your right toes up towards your left knee. Exhale, guiding the right knee over the left leg, with the toes pressing into the left leg. Move the right arm along the floor.

Move arm away from body

Lift right buttock from floor

Push right foot into back of left knee

Turn head to face right

Relax left foot

3 Exhale to rotate further, trying to take your right knee to the floor. Stretch your right arm out at 90 degrees, and turn your head right. Hold for up to ten breaths. Inhale to release.

4 Once back in the starting pose, repeat the exercise, this time bending the left leg. Once completed, inhale and gently reverse the movements.

Turn head to face left

Hold thigh at 90° to torso

Left foot at back of right knee

Right arm guides left leg

Look straight ahead

Keep your back straight

CHAIR TWIST

79

Spinal twists such as this one are easy, effective ways to bring yoga into your day-to-day routine. The Chair Twist can be practised anywhere within a few minutes, as long as you have a chair with straight back. It is a good exercise for stretching the spine and releasing tension in the neck and shoulders. As with all yoga asanas, perform the exercise on both sides of the body.

1 Sit sideways on the chair, with the backrest next to your right arm and your feet on the floor. Place your hands on your thighs, and relax the shoulders.

Rotate shoulders

Keep feet planted

2 Turn right and take the backrest with both hands, inhale, and lift your chest. Exhale, twisting from the lower back towards the rear of the chair.

3 Stretching the spine up, turn the trunk, shoulders, neck, and head as far right as is comfortable, and raise your right arm. Hold for several breaths.

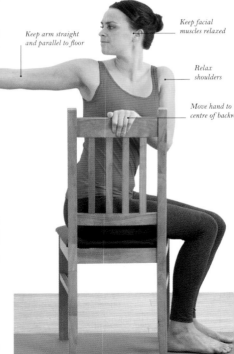

Keep arm straight and parallel to floor

Keep facial muscles relaxed

Relax shoulders

Move hand to centre of back

80 CROSSED LEG FORWARDS BEND

This pose is beneficial for the practitioner in several ways. Not only does it relieve tension in the lower back, but it also improves digestion and helps calm the mind. Additionally, it helps with the opening of the hips and outer thighs.

THINGS TO REMEMBER
When you are attempting to move your head closer to the floor, you may find that the front foot slips forwards. Counter this by sitting on a blanket, but with your feet on the mat. Be careful not to pull from the neck when you are lowering your head. The back, neck, and head should remain aligned, and you should keep your back straight throughout the entire exercise.

Align head to neck and back

Elongate your spine, keeping it straight throughout

Pull knees down

Place palms in front of you

1 Sit cross-legged and well rooted, with your right ankle in front of the left. Hinge forwards from the waist, setting your palms on the floor. Exhale and lean forwards.

2 Pushing down through your tailbone, stretch your torso and arms, moving your palms farther forwards. As you exhale, try to move farther still. Hold for five to ten breaths before releasing.

Keep shoulders relaxed

Root down through tailbone

Look down towards hands

Straighten your arms

POSES FOR BALANCE

81 ## HOW YOGA IMPROVES BALANCE

Asanas and breathing exercises help build core and overall muscular strength and flexibility. They also improve reflex responses while developing a calm, focused mind and profound bodily awareness. This all leads to better balance and poise, both physically and mentally. Balance is improved by working the body through a range of different postures. With consistent, mindful yoga practice, the body gradually becomes better poised. Combine your practice with meditation to balance yourself mentally as well as physically.

82 ## TREE POSE

This pose helps aid balance through concentration, by building strength and flexibility in the leg muscles. Start standing with the feet together, and inhale as you transfer your body weight on to your left foot.

Feel chest opening

Keep ribcage lengthened

Place right foot high up left leg

Pull abdomen in towards spine

Keep standing leg straight and firm

1 Bend the right knee and, using your right hand to position it as high as is comfortable, place your right foot on the inside of the left leg.

2 Push down through your left leg and breathe deeply, finding your point of balance. Inhale, and bring your hands to the prayer pose.

3 Fix your gaze straight ahead and, inhaling, extend your arms up, touching your palms together. Take a complete breath, then come out of the pose and repeat on the other side.

83 HALF LOTUS TREE

This hip-opening, standing posture requires you to use not strength but concentration and balancing skills.

Press palms together over head

1 Start with your feet together, and breathe in to transfer your weight to the right foot. Bend the left knee and raise the left foot. Draw your left foot as high up the right leg as you can.

Use right hand to draw left foot up if necessary

Activate leg muscles for extra stability

2 Balance yourself, then lift your arms. Press the palms together over your head, and extend and straighten your arms. Hold for five to ten breaths, then gently come out of the pose. Repeat with the right leg.

Press raised foot against standing leg

84 EAGLE

This asana helps strengthen the core and so promotes centring and alignment. The joints are nourished by increased blood flow.

Centre your head

Press palms together

Keep torso completely vertical

*right leg
nd left leg*

1 From a standing pose, bend your knees slightly and balance on the left foot. Cross the right thigh over your left, hooking the right foot behind it.

2 Lift your arms with the elbows bent. Wrap your right arm and hand under and around the left, pressing the palms together. Repeat on the right.

HALF SHOULDER STAND WITH WALL

85

Inverted asanas reverse the direction of blood flow, increasing the supply of blood to the face and brain, as well as to the heart and other organs. Such postures are particularly restorative. This pose is good for improving circulation.

Keep thighs slightly angled

Stabilize yourself by pushing feet into wall

Raise torso away from wall

Use hands to support your back

Straight legs, supported by wall

1 Place your mat at right angles to the wall. Put a folded blanket on top of it, with the fold next to the wall. Follow steps 1–3 of Tip 65, but end with your palms flat on the floor, next to the mat.

2 Bend your knees, so your feet are flat to the wall and shins parallel to the floor. Pushing off from your feet, raise your torso and place your hands on the small of your back.

Point left foot

Keep leg straight

Support weight with hands

3 Take the time to carefully adjust your position, with the aim of making your back as straight as possible. Then take the left leg from the wall and point it straight up.

Point both feet

Align knees to hips

Hold torso straight

4 Bring your right leg beside the left, adjusting your hands for extra support. Breathe. Reverse the steps until you are on your back with legs up the wall.

Roll over by rotating along lower back

5 As you exhale, bend your knees over the chest. Gently drop the legs sideways until your knees reach the floor. Rest for a few breaths, then sit up.

CAT BALANCE

86
Quite a lot of the yoga postures that are good for balance tend to start from a standing position. However, Cat Balance begins on the floor. Practise this asana to develop your core and strengthen your arms and legs. Repeat each step five times, alternating limbs.

Keep back flattened

1 Position yourself on all fours, with wrists directly below the shoulders and knees under the hips. Point your toes. Draw your navel towards the spine to flatten your back.

Arm should be in line with ear

Draw tailbone back

Hold raised arm straight

2 Inhale and raise your right arm while tightening the abdominal muscles. Keep your arm in line with the body. Exhale to lower the arm. Repeat with the left arm.

Keep raised leg as straight as you can

Back is held straight

3 Return to the starting pose. Inhale and pull in the abdomen as you raise and stretch your right leg, aligning it to your shoulders. Lower your leg as you exhale.

4 Return to your starting position. On the in breath, extend your left leg and right arm at the same time. Hold for five breaths.

Keep hips level

Point toes

Spread fingers to help support body weight

THE COOL-DOWN

87 IMPORTANCE OF THE COOL-DOWN
The cool-down after your yoga practice is an important component of the session, so be sure not to rush or skip it. It will calm your mind and relax your muscles, but it also allows your body to absorb the energy that has been released through the various yoga postures, thereby maximizing the value of the session.

88 PHYSICAL RELAXATION
Assume the Corpse Pose (see pp.66–67), then physically tense and relax all the muscles in your body, one body part at a time. Start at the toes and work your way up. Once you have finished, start at the toes again and mentally relax all those same muscles. Last of all, take a few moments to relax your mind.

Keep neck elongated

Hips open and fully relaxed

Keep feet apart and turned out

Arms should be at 45 degrees to your body

Backs of thighs make contact with mat

89 MENTAL RELAXATION
The yoga cool-down, or relaxation stage, is more of a mental exercise than a physical one. This is because it requires you to send mental messages to your body parts, instructing them to tense and relax. Once that is done, you finish the cool-down by relaxing your mind, too.

Take time to relax your mind

90 HOW LONG TO RELAX FOR?

Your end-of-session relaxation is based on the Corpse Pose, which should also be employed at the beginning of your yoga practice. Relax fully by resting in this position for at least five minutes.

Knees bent, with feet on the ground

91 ENDING YOUR COOL-DOWN

While in Corpse Pose, allow your breath to be full and easy. Wiggle the fingers and toes, gradually waking up the body. Bend your knees, keeping your feet on the ground. Draw the knees to your chest, hug them in, and gently roll from side to side. Roll on to one side and push yourself up into a seated position. End by bringing the hands to prayer pose.

92 CUPPING THE EYES

Just as it is important to warm up the eyes before your yoga session (see p.26), you should also take the time to cool them down after your practice.

1 Sitting comfortably, with your back straight, rub your hands together until they begin to warm up a little.

2 Close your eyes. Breathing easily, place your hands over your eyes for several minutes, completely obscuring your vision.

IMPORTANCE OF THE CORPSE POSE

93

The Corpse Pose is the ideal way to end your yoga sessions, as well as being a good start to your workouts. It allows the body the time to absorb all of the good muscle and mind work that has been done during your practice time, letting released energy flow freely and expelling waste products from the muscles. It helps you relax in preparation for the rest of your day.

CORPSE POSE

94

In this extended version of the classic Corpse Pose, the full length of the body is held in alignment and completely supported by the floor. This allows for deep relaxation in all of the muscles.

1 Lie with knees bent and feet flat on the floor. Interlock your fingers behind your head. Lift the head to look forward towards your knees.

Use hands to assist movement of head

Knees raised and slightly apart

2 Lie fully extended, with eyes closed if you wish. Starting from your feet, work up the body, breathing any tightness out of your muscles.

Relax all muscles

Let feet fall outwards

3 Inhale as you raise your right leg by about 30cm (1ft). Tense the right leg, keeping everything else relaxed. Hold, then lower and switch legs.

Focus on tension in leg

Hold leg tense for one breath

4 Arch the upper back to lift the chest, pulling the shoulder blades in. Keep the head and bottom on the floor. Hold for one breath, then release.

Arch upper back on inhalation

Point toes away

95 CORPSE POSE: ADDITIONAL RELAXATION

The following postures can be tagged on to your Corpse
Pose relaxation at the end of your yoga session, or you can
pick and choose the steps that you think would most benefit
you on any given day, focusing on the areas that feel most tense.

Keep head relaxed and centred   *Tightly clench fists*   *Relax feet*

1 Inhale, raising your arms by about 30cm (1ft). Tense both arms, making fists with your hands. Hold for one breath, and exhale to lower.

Stretch fingers apart   *Allow legs to be totally relaxed*

2 Inhale to raise both arms, palms up and fingers apart. Tense your arm muscles. Hold for one breath, then exhale as you take the arms back down.

Lift shoulders off floor   *Raise fists a little*

3 Clench your fists and breathe in as you hunch your shoulders up and raise your arms off the floor. Hold for one breath, then exhale to release.

Close eyes if preferred   *Keep feet loose and relaxed*

4 Lie completely relaxed. Free your mind of all worries. Each time you breathe out, focus on the tension leaving your body. Rest for a few minutes.

Support head with hands   *Stack legs one on top of the other*

5 At the end of your relaxation, bend your knees and roll to one side. Rest a while, then use the hands to push the upper body off the floor and into a kneeling position.

96 USING MEDITATION

Although meditation is perfectly suited to everyone, it is particularly beneficial for those who have busy lives, either because of stressful jobs or because of a vast array of family and household commitments. Meditation helps calm the overactive mind, thereby re-energizing you, increasing your stamina, and improving your powers of concentration. Through the regular use of meditation, it is within your grasp to create a sense of inner peace and have a clear mind.

97 WHAT IS MEDITATION?

A good way to grasp the real essence of true meditation is to consider a lake. Think about how you can clearly see the bottom of the lake when the surface is still. However, when there are a lot of waves, you are unable to see much below the surface at all. This is the perfect analogy for the mind: when your mind is still, you are better able to experience inner calm.

98 WHERE & WHEN TO MEDITATE

You are free to meditate wherever you are comfortable, but there are some considerations to bear in mind. If you choose to meditate indoors, pick a room that is warm, clutter-free, and away from distracting noises. If you go outside, find somewhere with as little activity as possible but where you are safe and able to relax fully. Meditation can be practised at any time of day or night, but it is easier to train your mind if you are able to set a regular time slot.

MEDITATING TOGETHER
You do not have to meditate alone. It can be done in pairs or even in larger groups. Mass meditations are often held around the world.

99 MEDITATION POSITION

To allow yourself to meditate correctly without any distractions it is important to take a comfortable sitting pose. Your legs should be crossed, and your spine should be straight. Keep your shoulders straight but relaxed. This is an easy, natural pose for children, but adults may require some assistance. If you feel any tension in your lower back, try sitting on the front edge of a cushion.

Keep shoulders straight but relaxed

Focus your mind

100 YOGIC BREATHING

Correct breathing is a key part of meditation and concentration. First, oxygenate your brain with 5 minutes of deep abdominal breathing. Next, slow down but still breathe rhythmically, in for 3 seconds, then out for 3 seconds.

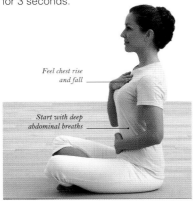

Feel chest rise and fall

Start with deep abdominal breaths

101 HAND POSITIONS

The hand positions shown below are all used in meditation. Make your hands as comfortable as you can; this helps you relax. Resting your hands on your knees or in your lap also helps keep the back and shoulders straight.

HANDS CUPPED
Place one hand on top of the other, palms up, and place them in your lap.

HANDS CLASPED
Interlock your fingers gently, and lay your hands in your lap.

CHIN MUDRA
Form a circle from your thumb and forefinger, and rest the hands on your knees.

INDEX

A

abdominal breathing 25
alcohol 12
aligning body 15
ankles, warming up 29
arms
Cat Balance 63
Chair Twist 58
Cow Arms 54
Downwards Facing Dog 37
Extended Side Stretch 38
Extended Sitting Stretch 49
Standing Arm Stretches 56
Sun Salutation 41–3

B

back *see* spine
balance 15, 60–3
Cat Balance 63
Eagle 61
Half Lotus Tree 61
Half Shoulder Stand with Wall 62
Tree Pose 60
breathing techniques 9
abdominal breathing 25
cool-down 65
inhaling and exhaling 25
stress relief 17
yogic breathing 69
Bridge Pose 46

C

calf muscles 32
Cat Balance 63
Cat Pose 50
Chair Twist 58
chairs, as props 24
children 16

Child's Pose 55
chin mudra 69
classes 19
clothes 21
Cobbler 47
Cobra 13, 41
cool-down 64–7
Corpse Pose 64, 65, 66–7
Cow Arms 54
Crossed Leg Forwards Bend 59
cupping eyes 65
cushions 24

D

diaries 22
diet 10, 12
doctors 20
Downwards Facing Dog 37

E

Eagle 61
Easy Floor Twist 13, 57
elderly people 17
equipment 21
exhaling 25
Extended Side Stretch 38
Extended Sitting Stretch 49
eyes
cupping 65
warming up 26

F G

feet, warming up 29
floor poses, props 24
food 10, 12
forwards bends
crossed leg 59
seated 52–3
standing 44
goals 22

H I J K

Half Lotus Tree 61
Half Shoulder Stand with Wall 62
Half Spinal Twist 13, 39
hamstrings 32, 53
hand positions, in meditation 69
health checks 20
hips
Cobbler 47
warming up 28
Horse 40
inhaling 25
joint problems 23
knees, warming up 28

L

legs
Cat Balance 63
Downwards Facing Dog 37
Eagle 61
Extended Side Stretch 38
Extended Sitting Stretch 49
Horse 40
Leg Raises 32
Legs Up the Wall Pose 45
Lunge Twist 51
Plank 31
Seated Forwards Bend 52–3
Sitting Forwards Stretch 48
Standing Forwards Bend 44
Sun Salutation 41–3
Tree Pose 60
warming up 28–9
Warrior 34

legs (continued)
  Warrior 2 36
  Warrior Lunge 35
Lotus Tree see Half Lotus
  Tree
lunges
  Lunge Twist 51
  Warrior Lunge 35

M

mats 21
meditation 10, 68–9
mental relaxation 64
monitoring progress 23
Mountain Pose 15, 30
muscles 30, 44

N

neck
  Plank 31
  warming up 26
nervous system 11

P

planning sessions 22
positive thinking 10
posture 14
practising yoga 18
pregnancy 16
props 23, 24

R

Rajasic foods 12
relaxation 9, 17, 54–9
  Chair Twist 58
  Child's Pose 55
  cool-down 64–5
  Corpse Pose 64, 65, 66–7
  Cow Arms 54
  Crossed Leg Forwards
    Bend 59
  Easy Floor Twist 57
  Standing Arm Stretches 56

S

Sattvic foods 12
Seated Forwards Bend 52–3
self-esteem 10
Shoulder Stand with Wall 62

shoulders, warming up 27
Side Stretch, Extended 38
simplifying poses 23
sitting positions
  Cobbler 47
  Extended Sitting Stretch
    49
  meditation 69
  Seated Forwards Bend
    52–3
  Sitting Forwards Stretch 48
smoking 12
spinal cord 14
spine
  abnormal curvature 14
  Bridge Pose 46
  Cat Pose 50
  Chair Twist 58
  Cobra 13, 41
  Crossed Leg Forwards
    Bend 59
  Downwards Facing Dog
    37
  Easy Floor Twist 57
  energizing 14
  Extended Side Stretch 38
  Extended Sitting Stretch
    49
  Half Spinal Twist 13, 39
  Lunge Twist 51
  Mountain Pose 15, 30
  Plank 31
  Seated Forwards Bend
    52–3
  Standing Forwards Bend
    44
  Sun Salutation 41–3
  Triangle 33
Standing Arm Stretches 56
Standing Forwards Bend 44
standing positions, props 24
straps 24
strength poses 30–43
stress relief 17
stretches
  Bridge Pose 46
  Cat Pose 50
  Child's Pose 55
  Cobbler 47

stretches (continued)
  Crossed Leg Forwards
    Bend 59
  Extended Side Stretch 38
  Extended Sitting Stretch
    49
  Lunge Twist 51
  Seated Forwards Bend
    52–3
  Sitting Forwards Stretch 48
  Standing Arm Stretches 56
  Standing Forwards Bend
    44
Sun Salutation 41–3

T

Tamasic foods 12
teachers 19
tension, checking for 20
tone, poses for 44–53
torso, warming up 27
toxins 11
Tree Pose 60
  Half Lotus Tree 61
Triangle 33
twists
  Chair Twist 58
  Easy Floor Twist 13, 57
  Half Spinal Twist 13, 39
  Lunge Twist 51
  warming up 27

V

vertebrae 13
vitality 11

W Y

warming up 26–9
Warrior 34
Warrior 2 36
Warrior Lunge 35
yogic breathing 69

ACKNOWLEDGMENTS

Sands Publishing Solutions would like to thank
Poggy Hatton for her efficient consultancy work during the project,
as well as for her assistance in fine-tuning the contents at the outset;
Natalie Godwin for design assistance; and the ever-brilliant Hilary Bird
for making such swift work of the index.

Dorling Kindersley would like to thank the following photographers:
Vanessa Davies, Guy Drayton, John Freeman, Steve Gorton, Sian Irvine,
Ruth Jenkinson, Dave King, Kellie Walsh, and Colin Walton.

All images © Dorling Kindersley.
For further information, see www.dkimages.com